Vagus Nerve Made Easy For Beginners

Leverage The Power Of An Activated Vagus Nerve To Fight Anxiety, Stress, Depression, PTSD, Trauma, Anger, Inflammation, Chronic Illness And More!

Wendy Johnson

Introduction

Did you know that the vagus nerve is the most important nerve you probably do not even know of? This nerve helps control numerous vital aspects of your physiology including the ability to speak, digestion, sweating, blood pressure and even heart rate. It is virtually found all over the body and even the slightest injury to this nerve could trigger an endless list of unpleasant symptoms such as chronic stress, anxiety, depression, tachycardia, difficulty in swallowing and speaking and even intestinal issues.

Fortunately, you can harness the power of your vagus nerve and keep it stimulated and engaged. However, you can only do that when you fully understand the incredible strength of your vagus nerve, and this is what this book will cover; everything you need to know about the vagus nerve, and how to use it to achieve overall general health and wellbeing.

Table of Contents

What Exactly Is The Vagus Nerve?

Let us first start our discussion by understanding what the vagus nerve is. Vagus is a Latin word that means, "to wander." Even the English words vagrant, vague and vagabond all come from the root word "vagus." The vagus nerve thus is known as the "wandering nerve". This is because it splits into multiple branches that diverge from two thick stems that are rooted in the brainstem and cerebellum. The vagus nerve then meanders into the lowest innards of your abdomen touching a host of major organs along the way.

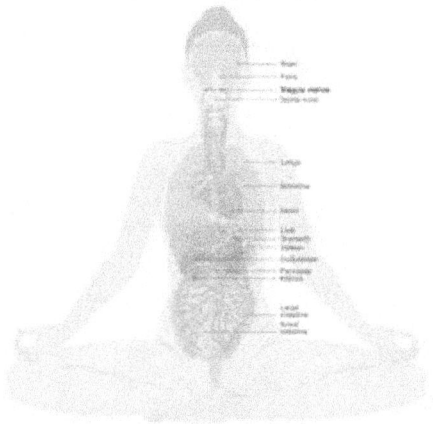

https://www.shutterstock.com/image-illustration/illustration-showing-vagus-nerve-meditaion-260nw-2058631652.jpg

The first person to note the vagus nerve and its role in social behavior was Sir Charles Darwin in his book 'The Expression of Emotions in Man and Animals' that was published in 1872. In the book, he proposed that the vagus nerve and the central nervous system engage in a reciprocal and dynamic exchange of neurologic information and this has an effect on the spontaneous expression of emotions. Sir Darwin asserts that human affective expression is integral to natural selection, adaptation, and survival.

Instead of simply being a reaction to the experience, Darwin hypothesized that the expression of emotions is linked reciprocally to physiology. He also hypothesized that distinct neural pathways exchange information bi-directionally between the brain structures and the major visceral organs such as the gut, lungs and the heart.

An excerpt of the book reads: "When the heart is affected it reacts on the brain; and the state of the brain again reacts through the pneumo-gastric (vagus) nerve on the heart; so that under any excitement there will be much mutual action and reaction between these, the two most important organs of the body (Darwin, 1872, page 69)." This only shows that Darwin's book was perhaps one of the first Western scientific

7

acknowledgments of the connection between the mind and the body.

The vagus nerve is the longest among the other 12 cranial nerves. 80% of the vagus nerve fibers i.e. 4 out of 5 pathways send information from your body to the brain, and when you hear someone tell you to "trust your gut," they are simply telling you to "trust your vagus nerve" in other words. Gut instincts and visceral feelings are literally emotional instincts transmitted up to your brain through the vagus nerve. The other fifth pathway is the only one that travels in the opposite direction sending signals from the brain to all parts of your body.

The vagus nerve is a long bundle of sensory and motor fibers that is anchored by your brain stem. It travels down through your neck and into the chest where it splits into the right vagus and left vagus to link your brain stem to the lungs, heart, and gut. It then branches farther along the way into tens of thousands of nerve fibers that interact with and touch the kidneys, tongue, ears, neck, female fertility organs, ureter, gallbladder, spleen, liver, and nearly every other organ.

The vagus nerve runs through the entire nervous system - your involuntary nerve center - and even controls all your unconscious bodily functions, in addition to functions such as sweating, breathing, food digestion and keeping your heart rate constant. Furthermore, it assists in controlling taste, stimulation of saliva production, the release of testosterone and bile juice, which plays a major role in producing orgasms and promoting fertility in women.

It also promotes the healthy functioning of the kidney and helps to regulate normal blood sugar balance and blood pressure. Indeed, without the vagus nerve, the key body functions that support your life would not be maintained.

The activity of the vagus nerve is known as the vagal tone and is measured by vis-à-vis RSA (respiratory sinus arrhythmia). RSA is a term used to describe the rhythmic decrease and increase of the heart rate, which occurs synchronously while you breathe. When you breathe in, your heart rate increases and vagal influence decreases (sympathetic nervous system influence increases). During breathing out, however, your heart rate decreases (parasympathetic nervous system influence) while your vagus influence increases. RSA is, therefore, an indicator of vagal tone that is used to examine the functional state of your parasympathetic nervous system.

In particular, the amplitude of the variability of RSA presents a measure of how the vagus nerve influences the heart.

Higher levels of RSA variability point out to a superior vagal tone during the breathing cycle, and this reflects your body's ability to respond to the ever-increasing environmental challenges and metabolic demands.

That said; the vagus nerve provides the primary control for your parasympathetic nervous system's response. When you are not in any danger or duress, the vagus nerve sends signals to the respective organs to slow breathing rates, slow the heart and increase digestion. However when under duress or stress, control shifts to the sympathetic nervous system, which produces the opposite effects. It is important to note that both of these systems cannot operate optimally at the same time.

The sympathetic nervous system's work is to fire you up like turning the key on a car's ignition and then rev you up. It flourishes on cortisol and adrenaline because it is part of the "fight or flight" response. On the other hand, the parasympathetic nervous system, is the exact opposite. It is set up to slow you down the same way brakes do to a moving vehicle. It uses neurotransmitters such as GABA and acetylcholine to literally slow down your blood pressure and heart rate.

With that understanding of the vagus nerve, let us now look at what happens to make the vagus nerve not function, as it should.

What Causes The Vagus Nerve To Malfunction?

When you are exposed to a stressful situation, your sympathetic nervous system is triggered. However, when the stress goes on or you are unable to switch off the physiological response that is triggering the tension, it will not take long before a few problems occur.

First, at the brain level, two pathways will be activated i.e. the brain intestine axis and the hypothalamus pituitary adrenal axis. Your brain will respond to this anxiety or stress by increasing the secretion of the Corticotrophin Releasing Factor (CRF) hormone, which goes through the hypothalamus to the pituitary gland to again stimulate the secretion of another hormone known as ACTH (Adreno-corticotropic hormone). The ACTH via the bloodstream finds its way to the adrenal glands and stimulates the production of adrenaline and cortisol.

Both these newly secreted hormones are introduced to act as inflammatory precursors and immune system suppressors. This could explain why you usually begin to feel ill when you are anxious or stressed and if this keeps up, you could ultimately end up developing depression, a mental disorder that is strongly linked to inflammatory brain response.

As if that is not bad enough, chronic anxiety and stress could cause an increase in glutamate levels in your brain. This is a neurotransmitter, which if produced in excess, further deepens the anxiety, depression and causes serious migraines. What is more, high levels of cortisol in the body shrink the volume of the hippocampus, the part of the brain, which is solely responsible for the creation of new memories.

In fact, since the vagus nerve is not capable of setting the relaxation signal in motion, the sympathetic nervous system stays active. This may make you suffer from anxiety, respond impulsively or experience disproportionate emotional responses. It is also worth noting that researchers from the University of Miami discovered that the vagal tone could also be transmitted from mother to child. An expectant mother who suffers from depression, anxiety or experiences rage and anger during pregnancy, the vagus nerve does not function as it should, and chances are that the child she delivers will have low levels of serotonin and dopamine and exhibit problems with the vagus nerve.

But, how can you know that the vagus nerve is not functioning as it should? Let us find out in the following chapter.

Symptoms Of Vagus Nerve Dysfunction

Dysfunction of the vagus nerve, when it is either underactive or overactive, can result in the manifestation of an extensive range of symptoms including the following:

Impaired Coughing

The afferent vagus nerve endings deeply innervate the larynx and pharynx airways to the level of terminal bronchioles, which extend to the lung parenchyma. They may also permeate into the esophagus and the external auditory meatus (i.e. around the Arnold nerve or the auricular branch of the vagus nerve). Sensory signals go through the superior laryngeal nerve and the vagus nerve to the "cough center," a section of the brainstem in the nucleus tractus solitaries.

The cough reflex comprises of a highly coordinated sequence of involuntary reflex muscular actions with the possibility for input of cortisol pathways also. The vocal cords adduct causing occlusion of the transient upper airways. The expiratory muscles then contract to produce a positive extreme intra-thoracic pressure of 300mmHg or more. This causes a rapid expiratory flow and a sudden release of the laryngeal contraction to generate an impaired and sustained cough.

15

Chronic Inflammation

In the body of a healthy human being, inflammation is a localized situation that ends on its own. However, if the innate immune response is disrupted, it could give rise to an incessant pro-inflammatory cytokine activity. This is especially true when the macrophages that are exposed to acetylcholine (the main parasympathetic neurotransmitter) are deactivated since parasympathetic hemorrhage from the vagus nerve hampers activation of macrophages.

This state of chronic inflammation underpins a wide range of diseases such as Alzheimer's disease, multiple sclerosis, inflammatory bowel disease, rheumatoid arthritis and possibly even sepsis.

Vitamin B12 Deficiency

A severe consequence of vagus nerve dysfunction or vagotomy (surgical removal of a portion of the vagus nerve) is a deficiency of vitamin B12. How is that so?

Part of the job of the vagus nerve is to arouse the parietal cells in the stomach to secrete **intrinsic factor** and acid. For the body to absorb vitamin B12, intrinsic factor is needed. Vagus nerve dysfunction inhibits the secretion of intrinsic factor, and that impairs the absorption of vitamin

16

B12. The deficiency of vitamin B12, if left untreated, could bring about dementia, nerve damage, and other health problems.

Vasovagal syncope

Syncope is the self-limited and spontaneous loss of consciousness, which is then followed by rapid and total recovery. The main trait of vasovagal syncope is an insufficient flow of blood to the brain, a condition known as **global cerebral hypo-perfusion**.

Do you ever faint after seeing something surprising such as blood or after standing for a long period of time or even after a long period of exposure to sunlight or heat? If yes, then your vagus nerve is partly to blame. This phenomenon, known as vasovagal syncope, takes place when your sympathetic division dilates blood vessels in your legs followed by an overreaction from your vagus nerve. Blood pressure drops and blood pools in the legs and without enough blood flowing to the brain, you momentarily lose consciousness.

The initiation of vasovagal syncope is characterized by a reflex activation that triggers a decrease in vascular tone and a rapid decline in heart rate. During the first few seconds of vasovagal syncope, you may see an empty heart on the echocardiography monitors due to the lack of preload in what is termed as an 'empty heart syndrome'.

Delayed Gastric Emptying

Also known as **gastroparesis**, delayed gastric emptying is usually caused by an underactive or damaged vagus nerve. One of the functions of the vagus nerve is to coordinate peristalsis. This is the relaxation and contraction of the intestine muscles to generate a wavelike movement that pushes food forward.

You will know that you are suffering from delayed gastric emptying if you experience spasms in the stomach, stomach pains, heartburn, nausea, and unexplained weight loss.

Dysphagia (Difficulty in Swallowing)

The vagus nerve's primary motor division is the **recurrent laryngeal nerve**. The recurrent laryngeal nerve is responsible for making a glottis closure possible when a cough reflex is underway and it produces the adduction of the vocal cord during bolus passage (food swallowing). If the recurrent laryngeal nerve is injured, you could suffer from a possible paralysis of the vocal cords. You could also suffer dysphagia (discomfort or difficulty when swallowing). Other symptoms include poor cough and weak voice.

Sustaining a vagal nerve injury near or at the base of the skull can cause a laryngopharyngeal deficit or a pharyngeal motor weakness, which could increase the risk of developing aspiration. Aspiration is the entry of bolus material into the lower respiratory tract or voice box from the gastrointestinal tract or the oropharynx.

Bradycardia

Bradycardia is a condition characterized by an **abnormally low heart rate**. It is a sign that there is too much vagal activity going on in your body. Technically, Bradycardia is defined as a low heart rate that is less than 60 beats per minute. However, marathon runners and long-distance athletes also have low heart rates but theirs is due to an adaptive increase in cardiovascular health and fitness.

An abnormally low heart rate could lead to a temporary loss of consciousness or even syncope. Bradycardia causes poor brain perfusion and inadequate cardiac output and these factors lead to fainting.

Anxiety and Depression

The link between anxiety and the vagus nerve is well documented (refer to the previous chapter). When the vagus is functioning properly, it opposes the fight or flight sympathetic response. However, a malfunctioning vagus nerve could leave the sympathetic system unopposed leading to an increased heart rate, insomnia and restlessness, anxiety, and hyper-arousal. Thus, normal vagal activity is required to keep the fight or flight responses in check.

A malfunctioning vagus nerve upsets your mood and can easily lead to depression. Depression is one of the most common mental illnesses and is characterized by a loss of interest in activities, fatigue, hopelessness and a profound feeling of sadness. The vagus nerve, which innervates the proximal colon and the upper gut has been implicated in depression and anxiety. However, the introduction of Lactobacillus rhamnosus into the gut causes a transformation in the expression of the GABA1b inhibitory neurotransmitter, which is associated with decreased levels of corticosteroids and ultimately a reduction in depressive and anxious behaviors.

Irritable Bowel Syndrome (IBS)

The dysregulation of the autonomic nervous system is a huge factor in the occurrence of irritable bowel syndrome. A Journal of Internal Medicine Study published in 2017 made a discovery that the vagus nerve is so closely entwined with the digestive system that its stimulation has the ability to improve irritable bowel syndrome.

IBS is characterized by altered bowel habits such as diarrhea, constipation, or a mixture of both, accompanied by abdominal discomfort or pain. Other symptoms of IBS include bloating. Visceral gut hypersensitivity and vagus nerve overactivity are believed to be a key factor in the development of pain caused by irritable bowel syndrome.

Weight Gain and Obesity

Many studies have found a link between decreased vagus nerve activity and weight gain. This makes a lot of sense given the fact that the vagus nerve regulates glucose homeostasis and the secretion of insulin. This means that the vagus nerve plays a key role in bringing satiety once you are full. Vagal afferents convey satiety signals from the gut to the brain and thus, the vagus nerve as it seems is an important component for keeping your appetite under check and helping to prevent the development of obesity.

The Polyvagal Theory

The polyvagal theory was developed by Dr. Stephen Porges as a result of extensive research which was meant to better understand the functioning of the autonomic nervous system and especially how it relates to post-traumatic stress disorder (PTSD) and trauma. In a nutshell, the polyvagal theory proposes that there are **three phylogenic and evolutionary stages** of the vagus nerve and that regulation of the different states of the nervous system is vital for the management of various mental health conditions.

The first stage, and this is evident in primitive life forms, is associated with immobilization behaviors such as feigning death or freezing when there is an actual threat. The 2nd stage entails the influence exerted by the sympathetic nervous system. This increases the metabolic output and holds back the vagal tone/parasympathetic nervous system to mobilize for the fight or flight. The third and last stage that is unique to all mammals involves the introduction of the myelinated vagal nerve, which is capable of regulating the cardiac output rapidly to facilitate disengagement and engagement from the environmental stimuli.

By now, you already know that the autonomic nervous system (ANS) is regulated by the tenth cranial nerve i.e. the vagus nerve. The vagus nerve connects the major systems to the brain and it, therefore, supports body-mind communications.

All mammals have 2 vagal circuits: the **dorsal vagal complex (DVC)**, which is the evolutionary older circuit and the **ventral vagal complex (VVC),** also known as the "social nervous system" which is a more recently evolved vagal circuit.

The social nervous system (ventral vagal) connects above your diaphragm to the facial muscles around your eyes and mouth, inner ear, pharynx, larynx, lungs, and the heart. The dorsal vagal complex, on the other hand, connects to the organs underneath your diaphragm. This includes the large and small intestines as well as the kidneys, liver, spleen and the stomach.

Generally speaking, the vagus nerve is at all times linked to the parasympathetic nervous system and has a calming influence upon the sympathetic nervous activity and notably, the heart. More importantly, Dr. Porges's research discovered that the parasympathetic nervous system is built upon two vital presentations, which depend upon whether you feel threatened or feel safe.

When you perceive the environment around you to be safe, the parasympathetic nervous system facilitates relaxation, digestion and rest. On the other hand, however, when you feel threatened, the parasympathetic nervous system has in place a defensive mode.

Bio-Behavioral Defenses of Your Parasympathetic Nervous System

When perceiving threat around you, the most obvious reaction is to attempt to engage the **ventral vagal complex** to restore back the sense of safety and connection. However, if you are still unable to create a safe and relational bond, you will gradually turn to older evolutionary behavioral defense strategies.

The first thing that is likely to happen is that you'll resort to the sympathetic nervous system actions such as the fight or flight to gather yourself together into self-protection. If the fight or flight is activated, you may begin to feel panicky, anxious or shaky.

However, if the sympathetic nervous system is deemed futile in its efforts to re-establish your safety, you will immediately draw upon your oldest evolutionary part of the vagus nerve i.e. the dorsal vagal complex (DVC). This more primitive approach takes on your parasympathetic nervous system in a crude way. At this point, your parasympathetic nervous system engages by immobilizing defensive strategies, which will result in either dissociation where you might feel dizzy, nauseated or tired, and in extreme cases, you may end up fainting.

The Polyvagal Brakes

Both the **ventral vagal complex (VVC)** and the **dorsal vagal complex (DVC)** make an effort to exert restraint on the sympathetic nervous system. Dr. Porges uses the figure of speech to suggest that the vagus nerve can be likened to pressing your foot down on the brake pedal when driving a vehicle to bring it to a halt.

The ventral vagal complex can be likened to a "refined brake" because it has a soothing and calming effect that is reflected in the variability of the heart rate rhythmic oscillations. On the other hand, the dorsal vagal defensive strategy can be likened to applying emergency abrupt vagal brakes and that is why being stuck in the dorsal vagal complex for a long time could have severe ramifications on your physical and mental well-being.

The Ventral Vagal Complex aka The Social Nervous System

Your ventral vagal complex is bolstered by myelination. Myelination is a lipid/fatty substance that wraps around nerve pathways to insulate them and intensify the speed at which electric impulses travel along the pathways. Myelination is increased through repeated use and result causes an increase in control or speed of learning.

Let's take for instance the myelination that takes place when you are learning a new piece of music that you will be playing on a flute. At first, you play the music notes carefully yet slowly but as you continue practicing, you will start to create seamless music, even without reading the music sheet at all.

These myelinated branches of your vagal system control your facial muscles that are associated with breathing, sucking, swallowing and even speaking. It also regulates the sympathetic nervous system pathways to the heart, and that is why they have the ability to rapidly initiate calm and relaxation.

Similarly, the pathways of the ventral vagal complex are strengthened through continuous practice. You will know that you are in your ventral vagal complex when you see a sparkle in your eyes or feel some warmth in your smile. You can engage your ventral vagal complex to relax or connect with others. If your anxiety is building up inside unnecessarily, you can use the ventral vagal complex to reassure yourself that you are safe. You can do this by engaging in strategies such as slow breathing and calm to help you relax or even scan around and listen for cues for safety.

The moment you realize that, you are safe; you will not need to focus outwards anymore. This will help to link you up to the restorative side of your social nervous system. In other words, your ventral vagal complex increases your ability to respond efficiently when you feel shut down with depression or when dealing with anxiety.

If you are feeling anxious, you are most likely to have activated a key defense reaction of the sympathetic nervous system i.e. the fight or flight. Sympathetic actions entail mobilization. This means that you have to move your body to release the buildup of the hormone cortisol. You can also engage your ventral vagal complex by vigorously rubbing your hands together and then physically touch your legs, arms, upper chest, neck and even your face. Alternatively, you can try out physical movements that feel safe like shaking your legs and arms to release stress or going for a walk. When you feel safe, you can engage your ventral vagal complex to use the energy of your sympathetic nervous system to play, laugh and dance.

On the contrary, feeling numb, depressed, or shut down is an indication that you have activated the defensive reactions of the parasympathetic nervous system and this is characterized by immobilization. If at any one time you have gone through a traumatic experience in your life, it could be possible that you are perceiving threats in your surroundings that are not even happening at that very moment. This happens because the most common symptom of Post Traumatic Stress Disorder is confusion between the present and the past.

In such a scenario, your ventral vagal complex can help you know that you are actually not in any imminent danger. This should allow you to access the relaxing positive element of the "rest and digest" elements of your parasympathetic nervous system. If possible, you can seek the loving connection of a caring partner, friend, family member or pet. At first, you may need to call someone you trust and listen to the sound of his or her voice. You could also visualize a protective friend or a loving pet just to restore that sense of connection.

Let us now learn how to stimulate the vagus nerve for it to function efficiently.

Vagus Nerve Stimulation

By stimulating your vagus nerve, your body releases a variety of enzymes and hormones such as oxytocin and acetylcholine, which help to keep your immune system in check. This will result in feelings of relaxation, improvements in memory and reduction in inflammation. Activation of the vagus nerve has also been shown to reduce tension headaches and allergic reactions.

Regulation of the nervous system depends on the goldilocks principle. For instance, you recognize that you are "***too cold***" when you are feeling hopeless, depressed or shut down. You are "***too hot***" when you feel panicky, irritable or anxious. Sometimes you even alternate between both states and you could liken that to driving a vehicle with one foot on the accelerator and the other foot on the brake pedal.

Exercises that regulate your vagus nerve are focused on either re-energizing or relaxing, and this hinges on what you need to feel 'just right' given the circumstances. In this chapter, we will cover some practices that control, influence or change the functioning of the vagus nerve through the body and mind feedback loop.

31

You can practice this exercise either in the office or in the comfort of your living room.

Diaphragmatic Breathing

You cannot consciously and directly stimulate your vagus nerve as you would with a device that runs on electricity. But, it is possible to stimulate your vagus nerve by getting into the rest-and-digest response.

Do you remember the parts of your body that the vagus nerve branches to? The abdominal organs, heart, lungs or your throat; which of these parts can you control. Of course, it is not possible to consciously control your small intestines, kidneys or even your heart. However, you can control, to a certain degree, the depth of your breathing as well as your larynx muscles (which close and open the vocal cords to control the pitch of your voice).

Branches of the vagus nerve happen to innervate with your lungs and the vocal cords, and so it would make a lot of sense that you exert some influence on those two key locations so as stimulate the vagus nerve to facilitate the parasympathetic response in your body. But first, we will focus on the breathing part.

It should not come as a surprise to you then that the most commonly used and suggested method to activate your parasympathetic system is diaphragmatic breathing. Let's look at it from this angle – the **fight-or-flight** response is characterized by fast but short breathing, which borders on hyperventilation since your airways open up wide such that you are basically gulping in the air. On the other hand, the **rest-and-digest** state is always characterized by relaxed and deep breathing because your airways constrict and thus need a bit more time for both inhaling and exhaling to get the same amount of air in.

This could also work the other way around. When you are in the relaxed rest-and-digest state but gulp in the air in, your brain will take it as an invitation to fight or flight; thus, if you are truly in the fight or flight state but try to slowly breath in and out, your brain will perceive this as an invitation to rest and digest.

How cool is that? However, not all parts of breathing are made equal. For instance, if you have stage fright and you are about to climb onto the stage and just before you do so you take a deep breath and hold it in for a few seconds before letting it out, it will probably not work for you.

You see, every time you breathe in, you somewhat activate your sympathetic response. Your vagus nerve is suppressed and your heart rate increases a bit. But now if you hold that air in your lungs, you will actually accentuate that response. The opposite is also true. Every time you breathe out, you somewhat activate the parasympathetic response. This means that your vagus nerve is stimulated and thus your heart rate decelerates a bit. But when you exhale and keep the air out for a few seconds, you are in fact consolidating your parasympathetic response.

All this just shows you why the relationship between various aspects of breathing is just as important as the depth of the breath itself, and this is exactly what the vagal tone is all about. It entails the variability between exhaling or inhaling and the heart rate. If that variability is big enough, you are going to have a higher vagal tone, which means that you are able to easily switch from the fight or flight response to the rest and digest mode or even vice versa. How easily you are able to do that will basically be reflecting how resilient you are.

In fact, vagal tone is congenital to some extent (You may have been born a 'half-full glass' person, meaning that you possess a high vagal tone) and to another extent, it can be acquired. So in theory, the level of your vagal tone is all about the relationship between the two parts of your breathing i.e. inhaling and exhaling.

This begs the question, "How can you affect that relationship so that your body may become more adept at shuffling between the parasympathetic and the sympathetic responses with less effort?" You can achieve this through the **yogic science of ratio**. Ratios, in this case, mean that you will work towards aiming to extend the length of all four parts of your breath i.e. inhale-hold after inhale-exhale after exhaling). There is also the aspect of altering their relationship with one another for the purposes of parasympathetic and sympathetic management.

At first, this science of ratio might seem confusing or complicated, but it doesn't need to be that way. Try to imagine your breath as a weighing scale with the inhaling part of the breath (inhaling and holding the breath) on the left side and then the exhaling part (exhaling then holding the breath out) on the right side of the scale.

If you wish to sustain stimulation of the vagus nerve and the parasympathetic response, you will have to gradually extend your exhale and briefly pause once the breath is out. It is actually that simple. The longer you **comfortably** increase the time to breathe out in relation to the breathing in, the better the parasympathetic effect will become. Just remember that taking a deep breath is still very important and thus you do not want to shorten the inhalation part so much. What is important is to ensure that you deepen the breath. The table below is a simple example of a breath ratio:

Inhale	Holding after inhale	Exhale	Holding after exhale
6	0	6	0
6	0	8	0
6	0	8	2 (adding a pause)
6	0	8	4 (lengthening the pause)
6	0	8	0 (to transition back to normal breathing

This table is an example of building a ratio. You can see how you should progressively extend the period of time of the parts of the breath that you are interested in extending. And when you look at the last ratio, which is 6:0:8:4, you will notice that the 'breathing in' part of the breath should be 6 seconds (i.e. 6 + 0 = 6) and the 'breathing out' part of the breath should be 12 seconds (i.e. 8 + 4 = 12). This makes the duration for breathing out to be twice as long as the breathing in. This should give more emphasis to the parasympathetic effect.

If you put this ratio work into practice, it will help stimulate your vagus nerve albeit on the short term (while you practice) and increase your vagal tone for the long term (if you do it consistently).

N.B:

Do not hold your breath for too long. It is more important to lengthen your inhalation and/or your exhalation.

Do not make your retention longer than your exhalation or your inhalation longer than your exhalation. This means that it is OK if your Inhalation +Retention > is longer than Exhalation

Never force your breath. Keep the flow of your breath smooth. If you notice that your breath is becoming jerky, then you are practicing diaphragmatic breathing beyond your capacity.

Singing

Did you know that the vagus nerve is connected to the muscles at the back of your throat, larynx (voice box) as well as your vocal cords? It is then no surprise that singing has been shown to increase vagal tone and HRV (Heart Rate Variability) in individuals according to one intriguing study on healthy 18 year olds. Heart Rate Variability is closely linked to higher parasympathetic (rest and digest) activity, better stress adaptation and resilience as well as relaxation.

The scientists who conducted this study discovered that upbeat energetic singing, hymn singing, mantra chanting and humming all increase the Heart Rate Variability in slightly different ways. They found that singing set off the work of a vagal pump by sending relaxing waves through a choir. Singing in unison, has also been shown to increase vagus nerve functionality and Heart Rate Variability.

Then again, the researchers of this study also hypothesized that singing energetically can activate both your vagus nerve and your sympathetic nervous system, which might help get you into a *flow state*. In addition, singing *'at the top of your lungs'* has also been shown to activate your vagus nerve by working the muscles in the back of your throat.

However, the above study only included 18 year olds and no other similar studies have been carried out. That said, it is not yet clear how various types of chanting or singing could affect the vagus nerve in people of other ages or those suffering from mental health issues. For that reason, more studies are needed.

There is still yet another study that is somewhat similar to the one mentioned above where singing was found to increase the production of the hormone oxytocin both in amateur and professional singers.

Both sets of singers recall feeling 'energized' after a singing session although the amateur group had less arousal but experienced a greater sense of wellbeing than their professional counterparts experienced. The researchers point out that the explanation for this could be because amateur singers approached the practice as a self-realization and relaxation technique while the pros were achievement oriented.

This shows that if you want to stimulate your vagus nerve using this method, you ought to express yourself and try to

39

relax as much as you can while chanting or singing. Try as much as possible not to think about how good or bad your voice sounds or whether you will achieve the milestones you had set for that particular singing session.

Laugh More

Whoever said that *'laughter is the best medicine'* clearly knew what he was talking about and there is overwhelming evidence that highlights the major health benefits of a good laughter. And indeed, laughing can also stimulate your vagus nerve. A study found that laughter could increase your Heart Rate Variability.

Many centuries ago, Indian yogis instinctively struck upon the psychological and physiological benefits of self-initiated and spontaneous laughter, which they named *Hasya yoga*. The basic principle of Hasya yoga is that voluntary simulated laughter that is done within a group of people can rapidly turn into contagious genuine laughter.

The benefits of laughter are said to be entrenched in your nervous system. When you put the cart before your horse by voluntarily simulating your laughter, you take advantage of your intrinsic feedback loop. Any kind of laughter; be it voluntary or involuntary activates diaphragmatic breathing which triggers the parasympathetic nervous system and stimulates the "tend and befriend" response which is associated with a healthy tone in your vagus nerve. About 10 minutes of a good laughter is adequate to stimulate a wide range of physical and mental health benefits.

In the 1970s, a scientist by the name Norman Cousins wrote a book called *Anatomy of an Illness as Perceived by the Patient: Reflections on Healing.* This is one of the first books, which sold the idea of the association between laughter and well-being with the mainstream audience. Norman Cousins' interest was doing science based on empirical research on the neurobiology of emotions, which he conducted in his laboratory and he won many plaudits after some firsthand accounts of healing himself from what was perceived to be a terminal disease surfaced. He managed to cure himself by forcing himself to laugh and having a sense of humor.

In the early 1970s, Cousins was struck down by the sudden onset of a crippling and unidentified illness. However, he managed to regain his health by means of a prescriptive use of laughter as a therapy. This is how he recalls the manner in which he fumbled upon the health benefits of laughter:

41

"I made the joyous discovery that ten minutes of genuine belly laughter had an anesthetic effect and would give me at least two hours of pain-free sleep. When the pain killing effect of the laughter wore off, I would switch on the motion picture projector again (to watch Marx Brothers movies) and not infrequently, it would lead to another pain free interval."

A study that was conducted in September 2016 is one that has assessed the potential of stimulated laughter to enhance overall health. The study is founded on the hypothesis that your body cannot differentiate between laughter resulting from something that is genuinely funny and laughter that has been simulated. In other words, laughter which is self-initiated (such as watching slapstick comedy or practicing Hasya yoga) or spontaneous laughter, both bring forth great health benefits.

Cold Therapy

Studies show that when you expose your body to cold temperatures and your body adjusts to such, your sympathetic nervous system (fight or flight) drops and your parasympathetic nervous system (rest and digest) which is modulated by your vagus nerve increases. This turns on the immune system and stimulates the motility of the intestines as well as the reduction of heart rate. For purposes of this study, the temperatures suitable for cold therapy are up to 10°C (50°C).

Try to finish your next shower with at least half a minute of cold water and then note how it feels. You can then work your way and increase the cold shower periods until you get used to it. It may seem painful at first but your body will soon adjust.

You can also immerse your face in cold water to begin with. You could do this by bending forward and dipping your face into a basin of cold water. You dip your head in the basin such that your eyes, forehead and at least two thirds of your cheeks are submerged.

Intermittent Fasting

Intermittent fasting is an eating pattern where you alternate between periods of eating and voluntary periods of fasting. Reduced caloric intake and intermittent fasting have been shown to increase heart rate variability and this is thought to be a marker in vagal tone. Scientific studies from some quarters claim that the vagus nerve may mediate a decrease in metabolism when you are in the fasted state.

What happens is that the vagus nerve detects a drop in blood sugar levels as well as a decline in chemical and mechanical stimuli from the gut. This results in an increase of vagus nerve impulses to the brain from the liver leading to a slowdown of your metabolic rate.

Apart from activating the vagus nerve, intermittent fasting and calorie restriction can also improve your health significantly, and it is therefore something you should think of trying out. There are a variety of ways to practice intermittent fasting. Decide which method best suits your schedule and lifestyle:

a)   **Eat stop eat -** This method of fasting involves fasting for a full 24 hours for 2 non-consecutive days every week. For example, assume that dinner is the last meal you had at exactly 9.00 p.m. fast overnight and the entire day that follows. That means skipping breakfast and lunch so that you may break your fast again at exactly 9:00 p.m.

b)   **The Leangains protocol also known as 16:8 diet -** The 16:8 dieting pattern is by far the most popular protocols and it comprises of fasting for 16 hours every day while your eating window being 8 hours. Most people prefer having dinner then not eating overnight until the next day at around noon.

c)   **The warrior diet -** This method of fasting involves fasting during the better part of the day, then squeezing all your calories in the evening. Basically, this is a 20:4 hour split. 20 hours of fasting and 4 hours of feasting. The main aim here is to skip both breakfast and lunch then 'feast' on a huge dinner within a 4 hour window at the end of the day.

d)   **ADF - Alternate day fasting (fasting every other day)** - Just as the name suggests, you are required to alternate between one day of eating and then eating very little (caloric restriction) on the next day. On the fasting day, you need to consume 20% of your total daily energy expenditure. That makes it 400 and 500 calories for women and men respectively per day given that the recommended daily calorie intake is 2000 and 2500 respectively.

e)   **Spontaneous meal skipping -** Sometimes you just do not need to follow any structured intermittent fasting protocol to stimulate your vagus nerve. You may decide to miss some meals from time to time depending on the period that is convenient for you.

45

For example if you are too busy or if you are not hungry, then you do not have to bother yourself preparing or ordering food.

Probiotics

Probiotics are supplements and foods that contain live microorganisms whose purpose is to improve and maintain the normal micro flora (good bacteria) in your body. Probiotics are typically contained in high fiber foods such as sauerkraut, yogurt, artichokes, soybeans, garlic, onions, greens, bananas and whole grains just to mention a few.

As you may already know, Probiotics can help enhance your gut health. However, emerging research shows that Probiotics could indirectly improve your mental health as well. This is because scientists discovered that your brain and your gut are linked and this partnership is known as the gut-brain axis. These two entities are connected through the biochemical signaling between the central nervous system (the brain) and the enteric nervous system (which is the nervous system in the digestive tract). The primary connection of information between the gut and the brain is the vagus nerve.

Scientists have therefore branded the gut as a 'second brain' since it produces many neurotransmitters, which are similar to those that the brain does. Such include gamma-aminobutyric acid, dopamine and serotonin all of which play a key role in **regulating your mood**. In fact, it is estimated that about 90% of serotonin is produced in your digestive tract.

As such, whatever affects your brain often affects your gut and the opposite is true. For instance, if your brain senses danger around your immediate environment and initiates the fight-or-flight response, a warning signal is immediately sent to your gut. This could explain why you usually develop stomach upsets and other digestive problems whenever you find yourself in the heat of a stressful event. On the other hand, flares of gastrointestinal problems such as chronic constipation, Crohn's disease and irritable bowel syndrome could trigger psychiatric conditions such as depression, PTSD or anxiety.

How then does the vagus nerve fit in the gut-brain axis? Since it serves as the chief link between the brain and the gut, the vagus nerve is thus a modulator of the psychiatric conditions listed above, which are increasingly being linked to inflammation and gastrointestinal problems.

Stimulating your vagus nerve by consuming plenty of Probiotics can modulate the metabolism of monoamine by increasing the levels of dopamine, norepinephrine and serotonin. It also reduces the corticotrophin-releasing hormone to modulate the HPA (hypothalamus, pituitary gland and adrenal gland) axis. Together, all these processes positively affect your psychological state and uplift your mood.

The micro biota in your gut has a major effect over the activity of your vagus nerve as it works through the metabolic and neuroendocrine mechanisms. There are a number of studies, which have centered upon the effects of particular Probiotic strains for the purposes of improving psychiatric conditions and general mood. For instance, *lactobacillus rhamnosus*, a common lactic acid bacterium, was found to alter GABAAά2 and GABAβ1b mRNA expression to battle any GABA (gamma aminobutyric acid) changes that are implicated in the pathophysiology of depression and anxiety.

Another Probiotic strain *L. rhamnosus* was shown to decrease stress-induced corticosterone and this resulted in an improvement in depression and anxiety related behavior. It is therefore important to note that all these positive interactions between the brain and lactic acid bacteria **only take place in the vagus nerve**.

Neuroactive bacteria such as *B. longum* and *L. Rhamnosus* target the afferent neurons of the vagus nerve to initiate the transmission of microbial messages to the brain. The vagus nerve has 20% of efferent fibers and 80% of afferent fibers. A healthy micro biota secretes abundant amounts of short chain fatty acids including butyric acid, which stimulates the active afferent vagal terminals directly and initiates the relaying of messages from your gut to your brain. Nonetheless, it is not only the live bacterial organisms, which stimulate the vagus nerve. And this is proven by *B. fraglis*, a polysaccharide that is lipid free and one that is sufficient and necessary for the activation of the vagal afferent neurons.

Psychiatric conditions such as anxiety and depression are continuing to plague a huge chunk of our population and the most common and default treatment is pharmaceutical drugs, which have some serious side effects. But as scientists continue to unravel the mysteries of the vagus nerve, they are constantly discovering new information about how the vagus nerve is rapidly becoming an important contributor to a majority of the underlying neuro-hormonal and metabolic disorders associated with cognitive and mood functions.

Now, the attention is moving towards how health professionals can optimize vagal activity as a foundational solution to many of the rampant health conditions. Further, recent scientific research is pointing to a strong connection between the gut micro biome and mental health. This is making us understand that the micro biome could be the key for optimizing vagal activity and thus improving conditions such as anxiety, depression among other common psychiatric conditions.

How to Use Yoga to Have Control over your Vagus Nerve

Yoga is one of the widely used and most effective mind-body practices today. Yoga focuses on mainly movement sequences and physical postures. Historically, the term yoga has always been known for generations to describe yoga as a methodology (method of the given sets of practices) and yoga as a state of being (the goal or aim that such practices seek to fulfill).

The reciprocal correlation through which the neural platforms and the poses influence one another presents you with a lens through which the practice of yoga can help heal pain, facilitate resilience, and regulate integrated and systemic physiological systems.

It is important to note that you need to practice yoga as a cohesive system with all its Niyama/yama (ethical principles), meditation, Pranayama (breathing) and asana (movement) all included. Doing so will ensure that the somatic-focused (bottom-up) and neurocognitive-focused (Top-down) processes are combined. When you practice yoga as a comprehensive system, you will influence both the

51

neural platforms and the gunas for a synchronized effect on your behavioral, psychological and physiological wellbeing.

As such, it is worth noting that you should never break yoga practices apart where you focus only on one aspect such as Pranayama to down regulate your autonomic nervous system and neglect the other three. Instead, combine all four practices for maximum optimization of the relationships within the neural platforms and the gunas to create a stronger therapeutic container to bring forth the entire spectrum.

Let us start with meditation:

1. Meditation

Meditation is an awareness-building practice that involves one or more of either exercise of prosody, visualizations, chanting for vocal toning, mantras and affirmations. All these are used to support states of eudaimonia, equanimity and calmness.

Just as all other meditation practices, this particular one is also done with someone seated upright and the eyes closed. You should then recite the mantra silently in your mind. Some people recite the mantra in light and soft whispers to help with concentration. The following are some of the most commonly used mantras from the Buddhist and Hindu cultures:

- So-ham

- Om

- Ham

- Yam

- Rama

As you recite the mantra repeatedly, it creates a mental vibration, which enables you to experience a deeper level of awareness. As you continue meditating, you will notice the mantra becoming more and more indistinct and abstract to a point where you are led into a field of 'pure consciousness' from which the vibration began. As the practice deepens, you may feel as though the mantra is continuing by itself like the humming of the mind. In some cases, the mantra may even disappear leaving you in a very deep state of inner peace and calm.

It doesn't matter whether you are reciting or listening to the mantra; just ensure that your mind is actively focusing on every repetition. Each repetition is supposed to be new, fresh and full of life and awareness. Unite the mantra with your mind totally. Let them become one. Every ounce of your attention should completely engage with it. To achieve this, you should put some feelings such as gratitude, reverence, curiosity and care into practice

Repeating the mantra will enable you to disconnect yourself from the negative or unnecessary thoughts that are taking over your mind. This is because mantras are some sort of ancient power phrases with subtle intentions that enable you to connect with your spirit.

2. Pranayama

Pranayama is basically a term in yoga that is used to describe breathing techniques. Pranayama have been found to facilitate and control the ventral vagal complex of the heart while also aiding in the activation of the parasympathetic nervous system. It down-regulates the autonomic nervous system to promote the Sattvic foundations/ventral vagal complex in addition to widening the range of the safe mobilization to immobilization. Here are a few examples of Pranayama:

a) Bhramari Pranayama (The Humming Bee Breathing Method)

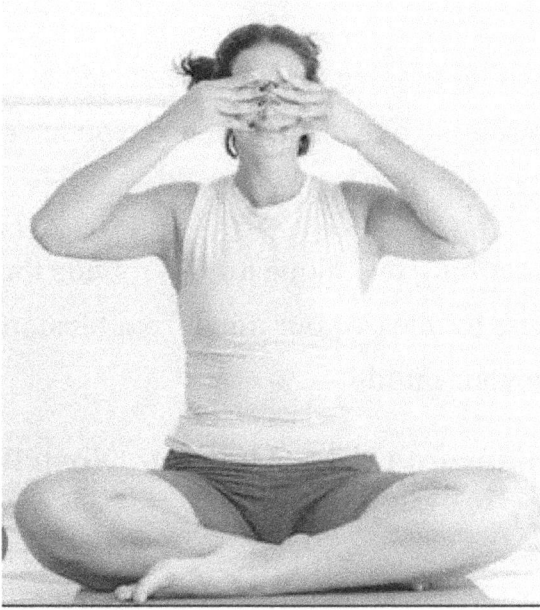

https://www.shutterstock.com/image-photo/caucasian-girl-doing-bhramari-pranayama-600nw-2253260545.jpg

- Sit comfortably with your legs crossed, eyes closed and your spine in an upright position. You can also lie on your back as you practice this technique. Make sure you are seated in a quiet and peaceful place.

- Place your index fingers against the cartilage in both ears

- Breathe in deeply and then press your index fingers slightly against the cartilage in both ears before you breathe out.

- Now breathe out while making a loud high pitched humming sound to resemble one made by a bee. You have now completed a full round of Bhramari Pranayama.

- Repeat this simple breathing technique for 6-7 rounds for maximum effectiveness to release your mind from tension and anxiety and calm your mind.

b) Nadi Shodhan Pranayama (The Alternate Nostril Breathing Method)

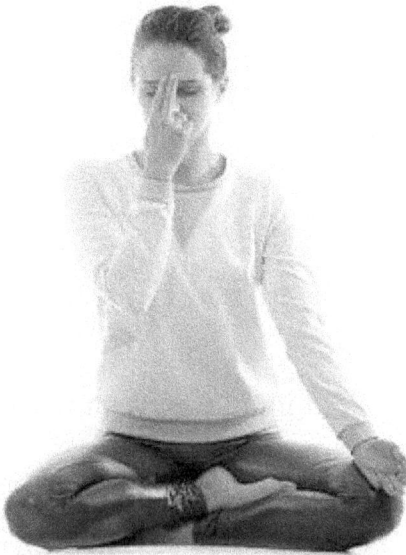

https://media.istockphoto.com/id/535514717/photo/yoga-practice-nadi-shodhana-pranayama.jpg?s=612x612&w=0&k=20&c=gqRlaHkQHBMN8A45U7028Ym8WewsFwGwFjsGb4laC58=

- Sit comfortably with your legs crossed and your spine in an upright position. Place your left hand on your left knee with the open palm facing up and close your eyes.

- Gently position the tips of your middle and the index fingers between your eyebrows. Place the little and the ring fingers on your left nostril. These two fingers will be used to close and open the left nostril while your thumb will close and open the right nostril.

- With those fingers in position, close the right nostril with your thumb by pressing against it and exhale softly through your left nostril.

- Inhale using the left nostril and close it by pressing the ring and little fingers against it. Take the right thumb away from the right nostril to open it and exhale through it.

- Now inhale using the right nostril and exhale through the left nostril to complete a full round of Nadi Shodhan Pranayama. For this method to be effective enough to help you, make sure you complete up to 9 full rounds. Remember the rule is to inhale using the nostril you used to exhale air from.

c) Bhastrika Pranayama (Bellow's Breath)

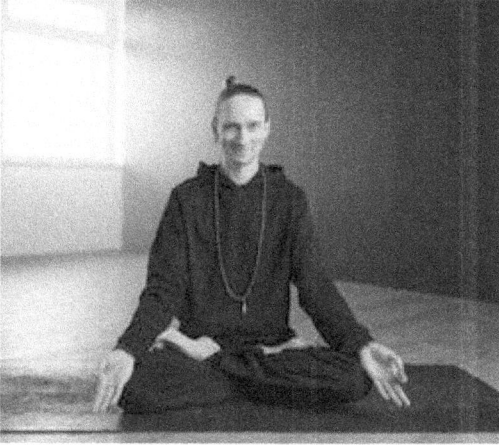

https://www.shutterstock.com/image-photo/yogi-man-sits-on-mat-260nw-2111042630.jpg

- Sit comfortably with your legs crossed, eyes closed and your spine in an upright position.

- Close your mouth and keep your body erect.

- Breathe in and out in rapid succession. As you do this, you will produce a hissing sound.

- Begin with about 10 exhalations and inhalations for every round. You can then increase this number over time.

- Some people do this exercise while combining it with Kumbhaka (holding the last breath). If you want to attempt this, breathe in deeply after the final exhalation then hold the breath in for as long as you can. You can now breathe out and resume normal breathing to mark the end of one round.

- There is also another variation of practicing Bhastrika. At the end of the last exhalation, you should breathe in through the right nostril and then hold your breath after a few seconds, breathe out through the left nostril.

- To complete a session of Bhastrika, do three rounds and make sure to rest in between the rounds until you can breathe normally. However, if you have limited time, have only one round and it will be enough to maintain your fitness.

- Have at least two sessions, one in the morning and the other in the evening.

d) Sheetkari Pranayama (The Hissing Breath)

- Sit comfortably with your legs crossed, eyes closed and your spine in an upright position.

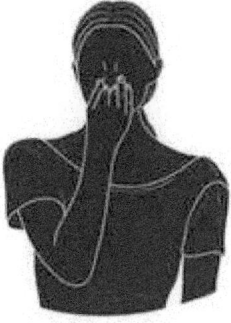

https://www.shutterstock.com/image-vector/alternate-nostril-breathing-nadi-shodhana-260nw-1215867820.jpg

- Roll your tongue upwards such that the lower part of your tongue makes contact with the upper palate.

- Pull your lips apart to expose your teeth then clench your teeth.

- Inhale slowly such that you first fill your abdomen, then chest and eventually your neck area to complete one yogi breath.

- As you breathe in you will notice that you will be producing a slight hissing sound, which will be almost similar to that of a hissing snake.

- Do a Jalandhara Bandha (chin lock) by bending your neck forward and then hold your breath for as long as you comfortably can.

- Let go of the chin lock while you breathe out slowly through the nose to complete one round of Sheetkari Pranayama.

e) Sheetali Pranayama (The Cooling Breath)

- Sit comfortably with your legs crossed, eyes closed and your spine in an upright position. Place your palms on your knees.

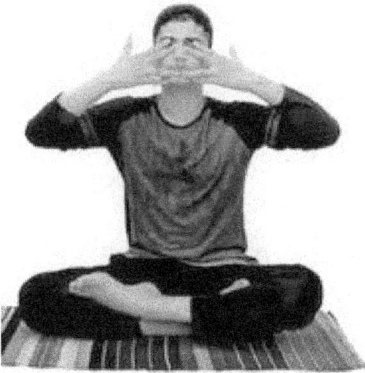

https://t4.ftcdn.net/jpg/03/01/04/99/360_F_301049969_1
KAw4zYcwlyqFNeCc8SJ73K9uH1oBiU2.jpg

- Roll your tongue so that it resembles the shape of a narrow tube. In other words, roll your tongue such that the left and right edges almost meet at the center of the top

- Slowly inhale and first fill your abdomen followed by the chest and lastly the neck area to complete one yogic breath.

- Pull your tongue inside your mouth and close your mouth.

- Do a Jalandhara Bandha (chin lock) by bending your neck forward and then hold your breath for as long as you comfortably can.

- Let go of the chin lock while you breathe out slowly through the nose to complete one round of Sheetali Pranayama. You can do as many repetitions as you want.

f) Kapalbhati Pranayama (Skull Shining Breath)

- You should do this on an empty stomach. It is advisable that you do it early in the morning before having breakfast. You can also practice it in the evening as long as there is a 4-hour gap since the last meal you ate.

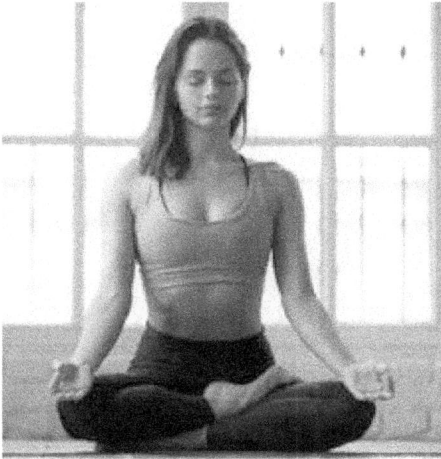

https://www.shutterstock.com/image-photo/young-sporty-attractive-woman-practicing-260nw-1223884600.jpg

- To do Kapalbhati, sit comfortably with your legs crossed and your spine in an upright position. Place your hands on your knees and relax your whole body.

- Inhale and exhale rapidly and ensure that the exhalation is more forceful while the breathing in is normal and passive.

- While breathing out, your belly should move inwards towards your thorax to help force out air from your lungs. You should be relaxed while breathing in to once more fill your lungs with fresh air.

- If you are a beginner, you can start with 10 or 11 repetitions, and as you get used to it, you will be able to comfortably complete 60 rounds in under a minute.

- After you have completed several repetitions, take a quick break until your breathing rate is normal. This may take half a minute to a minute.

- At first, you can repeat this process about three times.

Asana

Asana is used to refer to the gentle flowing sequences or restorative practices of yoga. Like the Pranayama, asanas help to down-regulate the autonomic nervous system. It is recommended that you work with a yoga therapist to tailor the best movements or postures that suit you and build your sattva and ventral vagal complex. When combined however, asana and Pranayama can help you cultivate sattva and ventral vagal complex states. In addition, they both build your ability to toggle between the various guna states and neural platforms by changing breath patterns and postures.

a. Balasana (The Child's Pose)

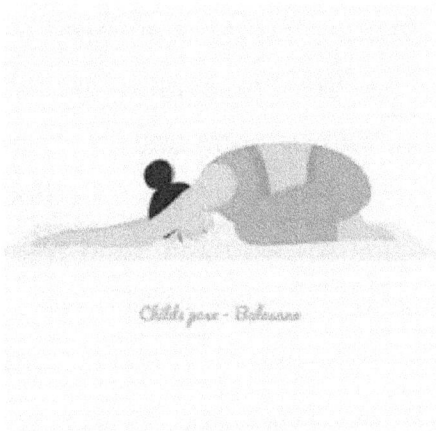

Child's pose - Balasana

https://www.shutterstock.com/image-vector/childs-pose-balasana-young-woman-260nw-1869040057.jpg

- Be on your knees and hands touching the ground.

- Spread your knees apart and let your big toes be in contact. Now rest your buttocks on your heels. If your hips are tight, you can keep thighs and knees together.

- Now sit up straight from there and extend your spine up through the crown of your head.

- Breathe out and lean forward as if draping your torso between your thighs. At this point, your chest should be rested on top of your thighs. Let your forehead touch the ground.

- Ensure your arms are extended and palms facing down. Press back slightly you're your hands to ensure your buttocks rest on your heels. Let your upper back broaden.

- Allow your lower back to relax and soften. This will make tension build up on the neck and arms to go away.

- With your eyes shut, keep your gaze drawn inwards. Hold the position for about a minute or even more if you are able

- To end the pose, use your hands to walk your upper body upright to sit back on your heels and get up.

b. Vrikshasana (The Tree Pose)

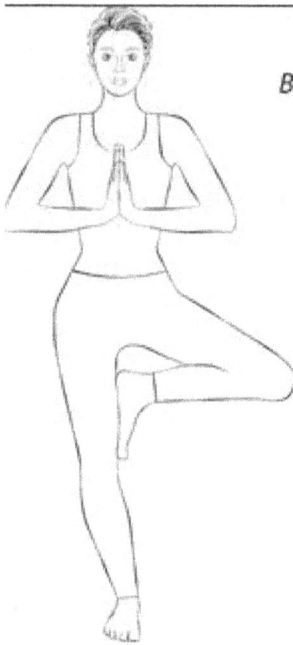

Tree pose
Vrikshasana
Bhagirathasana

https://www.shutterstock.com/image-vector/sketch-young-woman-doing-yoga-600nw-2380151939.jpg

- Stand straight and tall and place your hands on either side of your body.

- Bend the right knee and lift your right foot high up to be level with your left thigh. Ensure that your right foot's sole is flat and firmly near the root of your thigh.

- With the left leg perfectly straight try to find your balance.

- When you find your balance, inhale deeply and gracefully lift your hands over your head such that you bring your palms together in what is known as a 'namaste mudra' or the folded hands stance.

- Keep your back straight and ensure that whole body is taut the way a stretched elastic band is.

- Continue inhaling and exhaling deeply and slowly. As you breathe out, relax the body and as you breathe in remain taut.

- After a few minutes of this activity, breathe out slowly and bring your hands down and put your suspended leg down.

- Stand straight and stand tall as you did in the first step and repeat the pose with the left leg suspended this time.

c. Marjariasana (Cat Pose/ Cow Cat Pose)

- Begin by sitting in varjasana (the thunderbolt/ diamond pose) as shown in the image below.

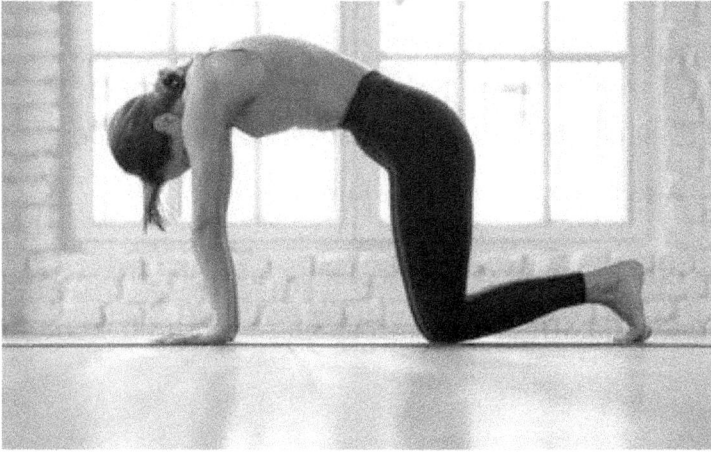

- Move upwards from that pose and make align your body parallel to the floor in a way that your body is over your palms and knees.

- While your palms are on the floor and positioned under your shoulders, your knees should be placed under your hips. Ensure that you slightly space out the knees so that your weight is evenly spread out. Keep your head straight.

- Breathe in deeply and push your back down as you lift your head to form a concave shape. Expand your abdomen as far out as you can to enable you to inhale the maximum amount of air.

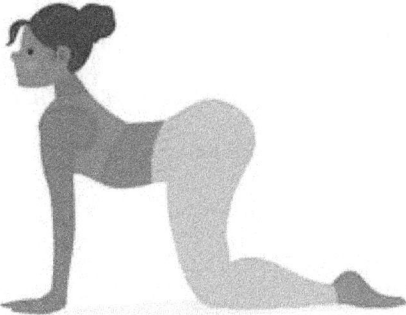

https://cdn3.vectorstock.com/i/1000x1000/38/42/cat-pose-marjariasana-yoga-young-woman-vector-35103842.jpg

- Maintain that posture for around 30 seconds as you hold your breath.

- Breathe out deeply, arch your back upwards while you hold your breath, and lower your head such that it is positioned between your hands. Keep your abdomen and buttocks firm until you feel the contraction.

- As you inhale deeply, maintain the pose for around half a minute then gradually work your way up to 60 to 90 seconds.

- Breathe out and slowly assume the Vajrasana once again. Rest for 15 seconds.

- For beginners, repeat the pose 10 times but then gradually increase to around 30 times. Relax for about 15 seconds before going for the next repetition.

d. Utrasana (Camel Hinge)

- Begin by sitting in varjasana (as shown in the previous image).

- Lift your body upwards away from your knees such that your knees now support your body.

- Your heels should be perpendicularly aligned to the ground.

- Breathe out deeply and bend your back backwards as you move your hands behind your body. Also attempt to hold your ankles one by one.

- Lean your head behind and keep stretching backwards until you feel a stretch in your belly.

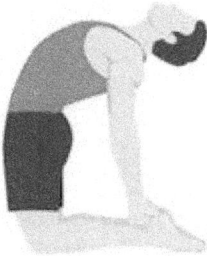

https://www.shutterstock.com/image-vector/man-doing-camel-pose-ustrasana-260nw-2200746009.jpg

- Maintain that stretch for about 20 or 30 seconds for starters but keep working your way up to about a minute or so. Do all this while you are breathing normally.

- Breathe out, come back to varjasana and relax.

- Repeat this pose 5 times at first then gradually increase to up to 30 times.

- Relax for about 15 seconds between each repetition.

e. Shavasana (Corpse Pose)

- After a rigorous yoga workout, this is the ideal pose to help you relax and rejuvenate your mind, body and spirit.

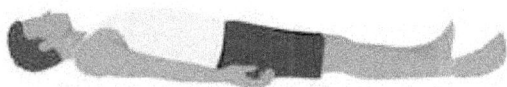

https://www.shutterstock.com/image-vector/man-doing-shavasana-corpse-pose-600nw-2294451195.jpg

- Lie down on your mat in a supine position.

- Stretch out your legs and keep your feet together.

- Let your hands rest on either side of your body, and close your eyes.

- Take slow but deep breaths and allow your body to completely calm down.

- Slowly scan your body from head to toe and identify any tightness, tension or contracted muscles. Consciously release any tensions that you find.

- Allow your body to move deeper into a state of complete relaxation.

- Stay in this pose for 5 to 15 minutes

- Once you feel totally relaxed, deepen your breath, bend your knees towards your chest and roll over to either side into a fetal pose. To release, breathe in slowly and rise into a seated position.

Niyama and Yama

Niyama and Yama are just but ethical intentions, which use attributes such as contentment, compassion and non-harming to strengthen your ventral vagal complex and sattva. By practicing Niyama and Yama, you create a foundation of restoration, connection, safety, peace and ease. You also learn to bring the experience of non-harming, patience and contentment to replace depression, anxiety, fear and pain by enacting compassion for yourself and others.

Metta meditation is a good example and it involves directing well wishes towards other people. First you need to direct loving and kindness toward yourself and thereafter, in a sequence of spreading out, towards somebody you already love, to somebody you are neutral towards then to somebody you have difficulties with and in the end towards everyone without distinction. Eventually, you can learn how to feel true compassion for even those that have hurt you very deeply.

Now imagine you are taking a walk down the street and you see and injured baby animal. Your first natural instinct would be to ease the suffering of the poor animal in any way you can think of. That warm sensation of compassion you would feel is loving kindness and the benefits of feeling that way towards yourself and others are endless. The more you practice loving kindness, the more you begin to focus on the positive in every situation.

So how do you practice it? The general idea is to sit comfortably, close your eyes, and imagine what you wish for your life. Come up with your desires in about three phrases. One phrase you can come up with could be "May I be happy."

1. Start by saying the phrases yourself: May I be happy.

2. Now say the same phrase to someone you appreciate or someone who may have helped at some point in your life.

3. Now, think about somebody you feel neutral about; people you neither like nor dislike. This one can be harder than you

think: It makes you realize how quick you are to judge someone as either negative or positive in your life.

4. Ironically, the next is easier: visualize the people you generally don't like or you are having a challenging time dealing with them.

5. Now direct the phrase to everyone universally: "May all beings everywhere be happy."

Conclusion

We have come to the end of the book. Thank you for reading and congratulations on reading until the end.

As you have learned, there is unbelievable power in the vagus nerve. Modern research has so far acknowledged the effects and role of yoga on the vagus nerve. The polyvagal theory has revealed the deep understanding of the complexity of the vagus nerve and the role it plays on the nervous system in response to stress and how we can use it to restore you to a place of optimal peace, growth and healing.

Now that you have a deep understanding about the vagus nerve and the physiological and neural substrates of your body and mind, you now hold the key to your healing and happiness. With such knowledge, you can now regulate your mind and emotions to positively affect your physical and mental health.

Finally, if you found the book valuable, can you recommend it to others? One way to do that is to post a review on Amazon.

www.ingramcontent.com/pod-product-compliance
Lightning Source LLC
Chambersburg PA
CBHW021526270326
41930CB00008B/1116